**The Everyday
101 Family-Fri(
Inspired by T**

by **Vesela Tabakova**
Text copyright(c)2014 Vesela Tabakova
All Rights Reserved

Table Of Contents

Delectable Gluten-Free Recipes to Help You Eat Well and Feel Great	6
Gluten-Free Salads and Appetizers	9
Avocado, Chickpea and Chicken Salad	10
Italian Chicken Salad	11
Balsamic Chicken and White Bean Salad	12
Bulgarian Chicken Salad	13
Chicken and Iceberg Lettuce Salad	14
Chicken and Avocado Salad	15
Greek Chicken Salad	16
Mediterranean Chicken and Quinoa Salad	17
Chicken and Green Pea Salad	18
Chicken, Broccoli and Cashew Salad	19
Warm Italian Beef and Spinach Salad	20
Beef, Lentil and Walnut Salad	21
Mediterranean Steak Salad	22
Mediterranean Beef Salad	23
Turkey Quinoa Salad	24
Tuna and Green Bean Salad	25
Tuna Salad	26
White Bean and Tuna Salad	27
Beetroot and Carrot Salad with Salmon and Egg	28
Salmon Quinoa Salad Recipe	29
Salmon, Avocado and Asparagus Salad	30
Potato, Pancetta and Asparagus Salad	31
Shepherds' Salad	33
Caprese Salad	34
Turkish Beet Salad with Yogurt	35
Mediterranean Buckwheat Salad	36
Greek Chickpea Salad	37
Bulgarian Green Salad	38
Okra Salad	39
Roasted Peppers with Garlic and Parsley	40
Gluten-Free Soups	41
Turkey and Quinoa Meatball Soup	42

Chicken and Buckwheat Soup	43
Greek Lemon Chicken Soup	44
Moroccan Chicken and Butternut Squash Soup	45
Brown Lentil and Beef Soup	46
Beef and Vegetable Soup	47
Beef and Vegetable Minestrone	48
Italian Meatball Soup	49
Meatball Soup	50
Lamb Soup	51
Buckwheat Fish Soup	53
Chilled Celery and Prawn Soup	54
Curried Lentil Soup	55
Lemon Artichoke Soup	56
Beetroot and Carrot Soup	57
Minted Pea Soup	58
Moroccan Lentil Soup	59
Spinach and Mushroom Soup	60
Broccoli and Potato Soup	61
Leek, Rice and Potato Soup	62
Bulgarian Potato Soup	63
Mediterranean Chickpea Soup	64
Carrot and Chickpea Soup	65
Roasted Red Pepper Soup	66
Spring Nettle Soup	67
Gazpacho	68
Cold Cucumber Soup	69
Gluten-Free Main Dishes	70
Mediterranean Chicken Casserole	71
Greek Chicken Casserole	72
Hunter Style Chicken	73
Chicken with Almonds and Prunes	74
Lemon Rosemary Chicken	75
Chicken with Almonds and Spinach	76
Moroccan Chicken Tagine	77
Mediterranean Chicken with Buckwheat	79
Chicken Moussaka	80

Chicken and Artichoke Rice	82
Easy Chicken Parmigiana	83
Sweet and Sour Sicilian Chicken	84
Mediterranean Beef Casserole	85
Ground Beef and Chickpea Casserole	86
Ground Beef and Rice Stuffed Peppers	87
Potato Moussaka	88
Eggplant Moussaka	90
Zucchini Moussaka	92
Mediterranean Lamb Casserole	93
Lamb and Potato Casserole	94
Spring Lamb Casserole	95
Mediterranean Pork Casserole	96
Pork and Mushroom Casserole	97
Pork and Rice Casserole	98
Pork Roast and Cabbage	99
Mediterranean Baked Fish	100
Sea Bass Baked with Fennel	101
Ratatouille	102
Spinach, Lentil and Quinoa Casserole	103
Eggplant Casserole	104
Eggplant and Chickpea Casserole	105
Green Pea and Mushroom Stew	106
Cabbage and Rice Stew	107
Rice with Leeks and Olives	108
Potato and Zucchini Bake	109
Okra and Tomato Casserole	110
Gluten-Free Breakfasts and Desserts	111
Winter Greens Smoothie	112
Pineapple Smoothie	113
Kiwi and Pear Smoothie	114
Quinoa Banana Pudding	115
Raisin Quinoa Breakfast	116
Berry Quinoa Breakfast	117
Baked Apples	118
Pumpkin with Dry Fruit	119

FREE BONUS RECIPES: Superfood Gluten-free and Vegan Smoothies for Vibrant Health and Easy Weight Loss	120
Peach and Cucumber Smoothie	121
Antioxidant Allium Smoothie	122
Strawberry and Asparagus Smoothie	123
Mango and Asparagus Smoothie	124
Pineapple and Asparagus Smoothie	125
Fennel and Kale Smoothie	126
Kids' Favorite Kale Smoothie	127
Kids' Favorite Spinach Smoothie	128
Paleo Mojito Smoothie	129
Winter Greens Smoothie	130
Delicious Kale Smoothie	131
Cherry Smoothie	132
Banana and Coconut Smoothie	133
Avocado and Pineapple Smoothie	134
Carrot and Mango Smoothie	135
Strawberry and Coconut Smoothie	136
Beautiful Skin Smoothie	137
About the Author	138

Delectable Gluten-Free Recipes
to Help You Eat Well and Feel Great

Gluten-free eating is becoming very popular around the world and there is a good reason for this. It is now widely recognized that products made of wheat are among the main reasons so many people are obese and there are so many modern day health disorders and complications.

Awareness of the negative health effects of gluten consumption has increased in the past few years and today surveys show that a third of Americans are actively trying to eliminate gluten from their diets. The main reason for this drastic change of dietary habits is that now we know that even without full-blown celiac disease we might experience adverse reactions to gluten. Gluten sensitivity, also called gluten intolerance, is a very real and common disorder. It is actually an auto-immune disease that creates inflammation throughout the body, with wide-ranging effects across all organ systems including our brain, heart, digestive tract, joints, and more. Gluten intolerance means having some sort of adverse reaction to gluten like bloating, stomach pain, constant fatigue, diarrhea or pain in the bones. All these symptoms disappear after eliminating gluten temporarily from your diet and then reappear when you reintroduce gluten.

People who have to follow a gluten-free diet for the first time are scared and confused because store bought gluten-free foods are often very expensive and really don't taste so good. They are hard to find and many people who have to avoid gluten feel overwhelmed and depressed by the fact that they have to follow this diet.

The truth is, learning to cook gluten-free is a challenge, but not an insurmountable one. The secret is that there is an easy and simple way to adhere to a gluten-free diet. All you have to do is focus on whole, naturally gluten-free foods. So much of the food we love is naturally gluten-free and, therefore, the safest and most nutritious way to follow a gluten-free diet is to cook at home and to stick primarily to fresh, unrefined and unprocessed ingredients. Fresh plain meat, poultry, and fish, whole eggs and plain cheeses, dairy based products such as milk, yogurt, sour cream and butter are safe if additive-free. Legumes, nuts, seeds, and plain tofu are great for vegetarians and, of course, so are vegetables and fruit. Gluten-free grain choices you can add to your new diet include rice, quinoa, corn, and buckwheat.

The Mediterranean Diet is a healthy, natural foods diet based on fresh vegetables, olive oil, lean meat, protein-rich legumes, and aromatic herbs and spices. Adopting a Mediterranean diet can be easy and cheap. One of its fundamental characteristics is that food is cooked using easily available ingredients - local, everyday products that we can buy around the corner or grow in our own backyard.

There are no processed foods with obscure and hidden additives therefore it is really easy to folloe a gluten-free diet without constantly worrying about it. And what's more, there are enough alternative whole grains like brown rice, buckwheat or amaranth that can be used in Mediterranean recipes to prepare healthy and delicious salads, soups and main dishes. Actually, almost any Mediterranean meal can be made in a gluten-free home; it just takes the willingness to try.

My gluten-free Mediterranean recipes are simple and easy to cook. I use a wide variety of brightly-hued vegetables such as red cabbage, eggplants, red bell peppers and tomatoes, carrots and squash, broccoli or spinach. I prepare only gluten-free whole grains, especially my personal favorites, quinoa and buckwheat. I never use thickeners for the sauces or the soups, and have discovered that meals can be as good and tasty without breadcrumbs or flour in the recipes. Although if you want to, you can buy ranges of pasta made from quinoa, brown rice or corn flour, I prefer sticking to a diet of unprocessed foods such as fish, meat, dairy and eggs, legumes or vegetables, so I didn't include pasta recipes in this cookbook. Instead you can enjoy my delicious alternative buckwheat and quinoa recipes.

The Mediterranean Diet is truly amazing and is really easy to make it part of a gluten-free lifestyle. You only have to be a little creative and will discover that there are endless food combinations and tasty, versatile, rich and healthy gluten-free meals for the whole family to enjoy!

Gluten-Free Salads and Appetizers

Avocado, Chickpea and Chicken Salad

Serves 4

Ingredients:

2 cups cooked chicken breasts

1 cup canned chickpeas, rinsed, drained

1 avocado, halved, peeled, thinly sliced

1 cup baby rocket leaves

1 small red onion, halved, thinly sliced

6-7 basil leaves, finely cut

1 garlic clove, crushed

1/2 tsp cumin

3 tbsp lemon juice

3 tbsp olive oil

Directions:

Place chicken, chickpeas, avocado, baby rocket, onion, and basil in a salad bowl.

Combine lemon juice, olive oil, garlic and cumin and drizzle over the salad. Toss to combine and serve.

Italian Chicken Salad

Serves 4

Ingredients:

2 chicken breasts, cooked and shredded

2 yellow or orange bell peppers, thinly sliced

1 small red onion, thinly sliced

1 small celery rib, chopped

1/4 cup slivered almonds, toasted

1 tbsp drained capers

juice of one lemon

1 tsp fresh thyme, minced

1/2 cup Parmesan cheese

3 tbsp olive oil

1 tbsp gluten-free mustard

salt and pepper, to taste

Directions:

Combine vegetables and chicken in a salad bowl.

Prepare the dressing by mixing olive oil, lemon juice, mustard, salt and black pepper. Drizzle over the salad, toss to combine and serve.

Balsamic Chicken and White Bean Salad

Serves 4-6

Ingredients:

1 lb skinless chicken breasts

1 cup canned white beans, drained

1 cup cherry tomatoes, halved

1 cup feta cheese, crumbled

1 cup rocket leaves

2 garlic cloves, crushed

1 tbsp honey

2 tbsp balsamic vinegar

3 tbsp olive oil

Directions:

Whisk garlic, honey and vinegar in a deep bowl. Add chicken breasts and turn to coat. Season with salt and black pepper to taste. Cover and marinate for thirty minutes.

Preheat a barbecue plate or char grill on high heat. Lightly brush chicken with oil and cook for two minutes each side or until golden. Reduce heat to medium-low and cook chicken for five minutes each side or until cooked through. Set aside in a plate, covered, for five minutes then slice.

Combine beans, tomatoes, feta cheese, rocket leaves and chicken in a salad bowl. Toss gently and serve.

Bulgarian Chicken Salad

Serves 4-6

Ingredients:

2 cups cooked chicken, chopped

2 hard boiled eggs, diced

2-3 pickled gherkins, chopped

1 large apple, peeled and diced

1/2 cup walnuts, toasted

2 tbsp lemon juice

2 tbsp olive oil

salt and pepper, to taste

Directions:

Bake walnuts in a single layer in a preheated to 400 F oven for three minutes, or until toasted and fragrant, stirring halfway through.

Mix together chicken, apple, eggs and gherkins in a salad bowl. Combine olive oil and lemon juice, salt and pepper to taste, and add to the chicken mixture. Sprinkle with walnuts and serve.

Chicken and Iceberg Lettuce Salad

Serves 6-7

Ingredients:

2 cups cooked chicken, coarsely chopped

1/2 head iceberg lettuce, halved and chopped

1 celery rib, chopped

1 big apple, peeled and chopped

1/2 red bell pepper, deseeded and chopped

9-10 green olives, pitted and halved

1 red onion, sliced

for the dressing:

2 tbsp olive oil

1 tbsp honey

2 tbsp lemon juice

salt and pepper, to taste

Directions:

Cut all the vegetables and toss them, together with the olives, in a large bowl. Chop the already cooked and cooled chicken into small pieces and add it to the salad.

Prepare the salad dressing in a separate smaller bowl by mixing together the olive oil, honey and lemon juice. Season with salt and pepper, to taste, and serve.

Chicken and Avocado Salad

Serves 4-6

Ingredients:

2 cups grilled skinless, boneless chicken breast, diced

2 avocados, peeled, pitted and diced

1 red onion, finely chopped

1/2 cup green olives, pitted

10 cherry tomatoes

2 tbsp lemon juice

3 tbsp olive oil

1 tsp dried oregano

salt and black pepper to taste

Directions:

In a medium bowl, combine the avocados, chicken, onion, and cherry tomatoes.

Season with oregano, salt and pepper to taste. Add in the olives, lemon juice and olive oil and toss lightly to coat.

Greek Chicken Salad

Serves 4

Ingredients:

4 small chicken breast halves

1/3 cup lemon juice

1-2 tsp chopped fresh rosemary

3 garlic cloves, crushed

1/4 cup olive oil

2 tomatoes, cut into thin wedges

1 small red onion, cut into thin wedges

1/4 cup black olives

3.5 oz feta, crumbled

1/4 cup parsley leaves, chopped

Directions:

Prepare the dressing from the lemon juice, garlic, rosemary and olive oil. Place the chicken breasts in a bowl with half the dressing. Stir well and marinate for at least fifteen minutes.

Heat a char-grill pan or non-stick frying pan over medium high heat. Cook the chicken for five minutes each side until golden and cooked through. Set aside, covered with foil.

Toss the tomatoes, onion, olives, feta and parsley in the remaining dressing. Slice the chicken thickly and add to the salad, then toss gently to combine.

Mediterranean Chicken and Quinoa Salad

Serves 6-8

Ingredients:

1 cup cooked quinoa

1 small roasted chicken, skin and bones removed, shredded

1 cup cherry tomatoes

1 cucumber, halved, sliced

1 red bell pepper, sliced

1 small red onion, sliced

1/3 cup fresh basil leaves, finely chopped

1/3 cup parsley leaves, finely chopped

1 cup black olives, pitted

1/3 cup pine nuts, toasted

for the dressing

1/3 cup red wine vinegar

1/4 cup olive oil

1 garlic clove, crushed

Directions:

Place quinoa, chicken, tomato, cucumber, bell pepper, onion, basil, parsley, olives and pine nuts in a large bowl.

Make the dressing by combining vinegar, oil, garlic and salt. Pour the dressing over the salad and toss to combine.

Chicken and Green Pea Salad

Serves 4

Ingredients:

2 cups chicken breasts, cooked and chopped

1 cup green peas, cooked or from a can

1 medium apple, diced

1 garlic clove, minced

2-3 green onions, finely cut

a bunch of fresh dill, finely cut

salt and ground black pepper, to taste

2 tbsp lemon juice

2 tbsp olive oil

Directions:

Combine all salad ingredients in a bowl and mix well.

Serve chilled.

Chicken, Broccoli and Cashew Salad

Serves 6

Ingredients:

1 lb fresh broccoli, cut in florets

1 cup grilled boneless chicken breast, diced

3.5 oz cashews, baked

3.5 oz sunflower seeds, salted and baked

2 tbsp Parmesan cheese, grated

1/2 cup fresh parsley leaves, finely cut

2 tbsp olive oil

2 tbsp lemon juice

Directions:

Wash broccoli and steam it for 5 minutes until just tender then transfer into a large salad bowl. Leave broccoli to cool and mix it with the chicken pieces.

Add in cashews, sunflower seeds and the finely cut parsley. In a smaller cup, mix the olive oil and lemon juice. Pour over the salad and serve sprinkled with Parmesan cheese.

Warm Italian Beef and Spinach Salad

Serves 6

Ingredients:

8 oz deli Italian roast beef, cut into 1/4 inch strips

1 red onion, sliced and separated into rings

2 tomatoes, sliced

1 red pepper, sliced

6 cups baby spinach leaves or fresh spinach, torn

2 tbsp olive oil

1/2 cup grated Parmesan cheese, to serve

for the dressing:

1/2 cup sour cream

1 tbsp gluten-free mustard

2 garlic cloves, crushed

Directions:

Stir together all dressing ingredients in a deep bowl and set aside.

Warm olive oil in a large skillet and sauté beef and onions. Cook for three minutes, stirring occasionally, over medium heat until beef is heated through.

Toss together beef, spinach, tomatoes, red pepper and dressing in a large salad bowl. Serve sprinkled with Parmesan cheese.

Beef, Lentil and Walnut Salad

Serves 6

Ingredients:

4 beef fillet steaks

1/3 cup olive oil

1 can lentils, rinsed and drained

1 bunch radishes, trimmed and thinly sliced

1/2 cup black olives, pitted

1 cup baby spinach leaves

1/2 cups walnuts, halved and toasted

2-3 green onions, chopped

1/4 cup red wine vinegar

1/2 tsp cumin

salt and black pepper, to taste

Directions:

Preheat a barbecue grill or char grill on medium-high heat. Brush steaks with olive oil. Season with salt and pepper to taste and cook for 3-4 minutes each side for medium or until cooked to your liking. Transfer to a plate, cover and set aside.

Put lentils, radishes, walnuts, green onions and baby spinach in a salad bowl. Prepare the dressing by mixing the remaining olive oil, red wine vinegar and cumin. Drizzle dressing over lentils mixture and toss to combine. Slice the beef and add on top of the salad.

Mediterranean Steak Salad

Serves 4

Ingredients:

1 lb boneless beef sirloin steak, about 1 inch thick

4 cups, romaine or rocket leaves

1 red onion, sliced and separated into rings

1 cup cherry tomatoes, halved

1/2 cup green olives, pitted

1/2 feta cheese, crumbled

1 tsp salt

1/2 tsp black pepper

for the dressing:

3 garlic cloves, crushed

5 tbsp olive oil

5 tbsp lemon juice

1 tsp lemon zest

1/2 tsp dried thyme

Directions:

Prepare the dressing by combining all ingredients in a bowl.

Heat a heavy skillet. Season steak with salt and ground black pepper. Cook it for 3-4 minutes on medium heat then turn it and cook for 3-4 minutes more. Transfer steak to a cutting board and leave it to cool. Slice it thinly.

Divide romaine lettuce among four plates. Top with sliced meat, red onion, tomatoes, olives and feta cheese. Drizzle with dressing.

Mediterranean Beef Salad

Serves 4

Ingredients:

8 oz roast beef, thinly sliced

6 cups mixed greens, torn

1 cucumber, cut

6-7 fresh mushrooms, thinly sliced

4 tbsp fresh basil leaves, torn

2 tbsp balsamic vinegar

4 tbsp olive oil

1 tsp salt

Directions:

Prepare the dressing by mixing vinegar, olive oil, crushed garlic, salt and basil leaves in a bowl.

Divide greens among four plates. Arrange beef with cucumbers and mushrooms on top. Drizzle with dressing and serve.

Turkey Quinoa Salad

Serves 6

Ingredients:

1 cup quinoa

2 cups water

1 cup skinless lean turkey breast, cooked, diced

1 small red onion, chopped

2 carrots, diced and cooked

1 cup green peas, cooked

2 tbsp olive oil

1 tbsp lemon juice

salt and black pepper, to taste

Directions:

Wash quinoa with lots of water. Strain it and cook it according to package directions. When ready, set aside in a large salad bowl and fluff with a fork. Add turkey, onion, carrots and green peas.

Combine oil, lemon juice, salt and pepper in a separate bowl and stir until well mixed. Pour dressing over quinoa mixture and stir again. Cover and chill until ready to serve.

Tuna and Green Bean Salad

Serves 4

Ingredients:

3 boiled potatoes, cut

9 oz green beans, trimmed and cut into 2 inch lengths

2 tomatoes, sliced

a bunch of baby rocket leaves

1 can tuna, drained and broken into big chunks

1/4 cup olive oil

2 tbsp lemon juice

3 tbsp homemade pesto

Directions:

Boil the green beans for 5-6 minutes. Drain and set aside to cool.

Prepare the dressing by combining together olive oil, lemon juice and pesto. Season with salt and black pepper to taste.

Combine potatoes, green beans, tomatoes, baby rocket, tuna and the dressing. Toss gently and serve.

Tuna Salad

Serves 4

Ingredients:

1 head green lettuce, washed and drained

1 cucumber, peeled and cut

1 can tuna, drained and broken into big chunks

1/2 cup sweet corn, from a can

a bunch of radishes

a bunch of green onions

juice of half lemon or 2 tbsp of white wine vinegar

3 tbsp olive oil

salt, to taste

Directions:

Cut the lettuce into thin strips. Slice the cucumber and the radishes as thinly as possible and chop the spring onions. Mix all the vegetables in a large bowl, add the tuna and the sweet corn and season with lemon juice, oil and salt to taste.

White Bean and Tuna Salad

Serves 4

Ingredients:

2 cups canned white beans, rinsed and drained

1 cup canned tuna, drained and broken into chunks

1 red onion, sliced

1/2 cup black olives, pitted and halved

juice of one lemon

1/2 cup fresh parsley leaves, chopped

1 tsp dried mint

salt and freshly ground black pepper, to taste

3 tbsp olive oil

Directions:

Put tuna chunks in a large bowl. Add the beans and gently stir to combine. Add olives, onions, parsley, mint, lemon juice and olive oil and mix to combine.

Season with salt and black pepper to taste. Serve chilled.

Beetroot and Carrot Salad with Salmon and Egg

Serves 4

Ingredients:

3 eggs, boiled and quartered

2 beets, peeled and coarsely grated

2 carrots, peeled and coarsely grated

5 oz smoked salmon, flaked

3-4 green onions, chopped

1 tbsp chia seeds

1/4 cup fresh lemon juice

2 tbsp olive oil

salt and black pepper, to taste

Directions:

Boil eggs over high heat for 5 minutes. Drain, cool and peel. Shred carrots and beets and divide them among serving plates. Cut each egg in quarters and place on top of the vegetables. Top with the salmon flakes.

Prepare the dressing by whisking lemon juice and oil in a small bowl. Season with salt and pepper and drizzle the dressing over the salad. Serve sprinkled with green onions.

Salmon Quinoa Salad Recipe

Serves 6-7

Ingredients:

1 cup quinoa

2 cups water

1 cup canned salmon pieces

1 red pepper, cut into strips

1/2 cup canned sweet corn, drained

1 tsp gluten-free mustard

1 tsp lemon juice

1 bunch green onions, chopped

3 tbsp fresh parsley leaves, finely cut

1 tbsp fresh dill, finely cut

freshly ground black pepper, to taste

Directions:

Rinse quinoa in a fine sieve under cold running water until the water runs clear. Put quinoa in a pot with two cups of water. Bring to a boil, then reduce heat, cover and simmer for fifteen minutes or until water is absorbed and quinoa is tender. Fluff quinoa with a fork and set aside to cool.

In a large bowl mix the salmon, corn, red pepper, mustard and lemon juice. Add in green onions, parsley and dill. Stir in the cooked quinoa. Season with freshly ground pepper to taste. Serve chilled.

Salmon, Avocado and Asparagus Salad

Serves 4

Ingredients:

1 cucumber, peeled and chopped

1 avocado, peeled and cubed

1 bunch asparagus, trimmed, cut into 2 inch lengths

1/2 cup soy sprouts, trimmed

1 can salmon, drained and broken into large chunks

2 tbsp light sour cream

1 tbsp lemon juice

1 tbsp dill, very finely chopped

Directions:

Cook asparagus in boiling salted water for one to two minutes or until bright green and tender. Drain and rinse and pat dry.

Place asparagus, cucumber, avocado, soy sprouts and salmon into a salad bowl. Toss well to combine.

Prepare the dressing by whisking together sour cream and lemon juice. Season with salt and pepper to taste. Drizzle salad with dressing, sprinkle with dill and serve

Potato, Pancetta and Asparagus Salad

Serves 6

Ingredients:

2 lbs spring potatoes, washed, peeled, halved lengthwise

4 tbsp olive oil

2 garlic cloves, crushed

6 slices mild pancetta

1 bunch asparagus, trimmed and cut diagonally into 2 inch lengths

1/2 cup green beans, cut into 2 inch lengths

1 tbsp red wine vinegar

2 tbsp olive oil

1 tbsp mustard

a bunch of green onions, finely cut

salt and black pepper, to taste

Directions:

Preheat oven to 350 F. Combine potatoes, olive oil and garlic in a large baking dish. Season with salt and pepper to taste and bake, turning occasionally, for about 20 minutes, or until golden.

Heat a large frying pan over medium heat. Cook the pancetta slices for 1 minute each side or until crisp. Drain and transfer to a plate.

Cook the asparagus and green beans in salted boiling water for 3 minutes or until bright green and tender crisp. Drain.

Break the pancetta into large pieces. Place in a large serving bowl together with the potatoes, asparagus, green beans and green onions.

Combine the remaining oil, vinegar and mustard in a small bowl. Season with salt and pepper and pour over the salad. Gently toss and serve.

Shepherds' Salad

Serves 6-8

Ingredients:

5-6 tomatoes, sliced

2 cucumbers, peeled and sliced

5-6 white mushrooms, sliced

2 red bell peppers, sliced

7 oz ham, diced

1 onion, sliced

3 eggs, hard boiled and sliced

7 oz feta cheese, grated

1/2 bunch parsley, finely cut

4 tbsp olive oil

1 tbsp red wine vinegar

1 tsp salt

20-30 black olives

Directions:

Slice the tomatoes, cut the cucumbers, peppers and onion, thinly slice the mushrooms. Dice the ham.

Combine all ingredients in a salad bowl and drizzle with olive oil and vinegar. Season with salt and mix well. Divide the salad in plates and sprinkle with feta cheese and parsley. Top with egg slices and olives. Serve chilled.

Caprese Salad

Serves 6

Ingredients:

4 tomatoes, sliced

5.5 oz mozzarella cheese, sliced

10 fresh basil leaves

3 tbsp olive oil

2 tbsp balsamic vinegar

salt, to taste

Directions:

Slice the tomatoes and mozzarella, then layer the tomato slices, whole fresh basil leaves and mozzarella slices on a plate.

Drizzle olive oil and balsamic vinegar over the salad and serve.

Turkish Beet Salad with Yogurt

Serves 4

Ingredients:

3 medium beet roots

1 cup strained yogurt

1 clove of garlic, minced

1 tsp white vinegar or lemon juice

1 tbsp olive oil

¼ tsp dried mint

½ tsp salt

Directions:

Wash the beets well, cut the stems, and steam in a pot or pan for 25-30 minutes or until cooked through

When they cool down, peel dry with paper towel. Grate beets and put them in a deep bowl. Add the other ingredients and toss. Serve cold.

Mediterranean Buckwheat Salad

Serves 4-5

Ingredients:

1 cup buckwheat groats

1 3/4 cups water

1 small red onion, finely chopped

½ cucumber, diced

1 cup cherry tomatoes, halved

1 yellow bell pepper, chopped

a bunch of parsley, finely cut

1 preserved lemon, finely chopped

1 cup chickpeas, cooked or canned, drained

juice of half lemon

1 tsp dried basil

2 tbsp olive oil

Directions:

Heat a large dry saucepan and toast the buckwheat for about three minutes. Boil the water and add it carefully to the buckwheat.

Cover, reduce heat and simmer until buckwheat is tender and all liquid is absorbed (5-7 minutes). Remove from heat, fluff with a fork and set aside to cool. Mix the buckwheat with the chopped onion, bell pepper, cucumber, cherry tomatoes, parsley, preserved lemon and chickpeas in a salad bowl.

Whisk the lemon juice with olive oil and basil, season with salt and pepper to taste, pour over the salad and stir. Serve at room temperature.

Greek Chickpea Salad

Serves 4

Ingredients:

1 cup canned chickpeas, drained and rinsed

1 spring onion, thinly sliced

1 small cucumber, diced

2 green peppers, diced

2 tomatoes, diced

2 tbsp chopped fresh parsley

1 tsp capers, drained and rinsed

juice of ½ a lemon

2 tsp olive oil

1 tsp balsamic vinegar

salt and pepper, to taste

a pinch of dried oregano

Directions:

In a medium bowl, toss together the chickpeas, spring onion, cucumber, green peppers, tomatoes, parsley, capers and lemon juice.

In a smaller bowl, stir together the remaining ingredients and pour over the chickpea salad. Toss well to coat and allow to marinate, stirring occasionally, for at least one hour before serving.

Bulgarian Green Salad

Serves 4

Ingredients:

1 green lettuce, washed and drained

1 cucumber, sliced

a bunch of radishes, sliced

a bunch of spring onions, finely cut

juice of half lemon or 2 tbsp of white wine vinegar

3 tbsp olive oil

salt to taste

Directions:

Cut the lettuce into thin strips. Slice the cucumber and the radishes as thinly as possible and chop the spring onions.

Mix all the salad ingredients in a large bowl, add the lemon juice and olive oil and season with salt to taste.

Okra Salad

Serves 4

Ingredients:

1.2 lb young okras

1 lemon

½ bunch parsley, chopped

2 tomatoes, sliced

3 tbsp sunflower oil

½ tsp black pepper

salt, to taste

Directions:

Trim okras, then wash and cook them in salted water until tender. Drain and let cool.

In a small bowl, mix well the lemon juice and sunflower oil, salt and black pepper.

Arrange okra and tomatoes in a bowl then pour over the dressing and sprinkle with chopped parsley.

Roasted Peppers with Garlic and Parsley

Serves 4-6

Ingredients:

2.25 lb red and green bell peppers

½ cup sunflower oil

1/3 cup white wine vinegar

3-4 cloves garlic, chopped

a bunch of fresh parsley

salt and pepper, to taste

Directions:

Grill the peppers or roast them in the oven at 480 F until the skins are a little burnt. Place the roasted peppers in a brown paper bag or a lidded container and leave covered for about 10 minutes. This makes it easier to peel them.

Peel the skins and remove the seeds. Cut the peppers into 1 inch strips lengthwise and layer them in a bowl.

Mix together the oil, vinegar, salt and pepper, chopped garlic and chopped parsley leaves. Pour over the peppers. Cover the roasted peppers and chill for an hour.

Gluten-Free Soups

Turkey and Quinoa Meatball Soup

Serves 5-6

Ingredients:

1 lb ground turkey

1 large egg

2 tbsp fresh parsley, finely chopped

1 medium onion, grated

salt and black pepper, to taste

5 cups gluten-free vegetable broth

1 medium carrot, chopped

1 onion, chopped

2 garlic cloves, chopped

1 green pepper, chopped

1 potato, peeled and cubed

1/3 cup quinoa, washed

Directions:

Combine the onion, egg, fresh parsley, salt and pepper in a large bowl and stir. Add in the ground turkey and mix with hands. Roll tablespoonfuls of the mixture into balls. Place on a large plate or baking sheet until ready to cook.

In a large saucepan over medium heat, heat the olive oil. Add carrot, onion and garlic and cook, stirring, for about 1 to 2 minutes. Add vegetable broth and bring to the boil. Add meatballs, potato, pepper and quinoa and simmer, uncovered, about 15 minutes. Season with salt and pepper. Serve with lemon juice.

Chicken and Buckwheat Soup

Serves 6-7

Ingredients:

2 lb chicken breasts

2-3 carrots, chopped

1 celery rib, chopped

1 onion, chopped

8 cups water

1/3 cup buckwheat groats

1/2 tsp salt

ground black pepper, to taste

lemon juice, to serve

fresh parsley, to serve

Directions:

Place chicken breasts in a soup pot. Add onion, carrots, celery, salt, pepper and water. Stir well and bring to a boil. Add buckwheat, stir, and reduce heat. Simmer for 30 minutes.

Remove chicken from pot and let it cool slightly. Shred it and return it to pot. Serve soup with lemon juice and sprinkled with fresh parsley.

Greek Lemon Chicken Soup

Serves 4

Ingredients:

2 lb chicken breast, diced

1/3 cup rice

2 cups gluten-free chicken broth

3 cups water

1 onion, finely cut

2 raw eggs

3 tbsp olive oil

1/2 cup fresh lemon juice

1 tbsp salt

1 tsp ground pepper

a bunch of fresh parsley for garnish, finely cut

Directions:

In a medium pot, heat the olive oil and sauté the onions until they are soft and translucent. Add the chicken broth and water together with the washed rice and bring everything to a boil. Reduce heat and simmer. When the rice is almost done, add the diced chicken breast to the pot. Let it cook for another five minutes, or until the chicken is cooked through.

Beat the eggs and lemon juice together in a separate bowl. Pour two cups of broth slowly into the egg mixture, whisking constantly. When all the broth is incorporated add this mixture to the chicken soup and stir well to blend. Do not boil any more. Season with salt and pepper and garnish with parsley. Serve hot.

Moroccan Chicken and Butternut Squash Soup

Serves 6-7

Ingredients:

3 skinless, boneless chicken thighs, cut into bite-sized pieces

1 big onion, chopped

1 zucchini, quartered lengthwise and sliced into 1/2-inch pieces

3 cups peeled butternut squash, cut in 1/2-inch pieces

2 tbsp tomato paste

5 cups gluten-free chicken broth

1/2 tsp ground cumin

1/4 tsp ground cinnamon

1 tsp paprika

1 tsp salt

2 tbsp fresh basil leaves, chopped

1 tbsp grated orange rind

3 tbsp olive oil

Directions:

Heat a soup pot over medium heat. Gently sauté onion, for 3-4 minutes, stirring occasionally. Add chicken pieces and cook for 4 minutes, until chicken is brown on all sides. Add cumin, cinnamon and paprika and stir well. Add butternut squash and tomato paste; stir again. Add chicken broth and bring to a boil, then reduce heat and simmer 10 minutes. Stir in salt and zucchini pieces; cook until squash is tender.

Remove pot from heat. Season with salt and pepper to taste. Stir in chopped basil and orange rind and serve.

Brown Lentil and Beef Soup

Serves 6

Ingredients:

1 lb ground beef

1 cup brown lentils

2 carrots, chopped

1 large onion, chopped

1 potato, cut into 1/2 inch cubes

4 garlic cloves, chopped

2 tomatoes, grated or pureed

5 cups water

1 tsp savory

1 tsp oregano

1 tsp paprika

2 tbsp olive oil

1 tsp salt

ground black pepper, to taste

Directions:

Heat olive oil in a large soup pot. Brown beef, breaking it up with a spoon. Add paprika and garlic and stir.

Add lentils, remaining vegetables, water and spice. Bring to a boil. Reduce heat to low and simmer, covered, for about an hour, or until lentils are tender. Stir occasionally.

Beef and Vegetable Soup

Serves 6-8

Ingredients:

2 lbs stewing beef

3 tbsp olive oil

1 large onion, chopped

1 cup mushrooms, chopped

2 carrots, chopped

1 celery rib, chopped

6 cups water

2 tbsp tomato paste

1/2 cup parsley, chopped

salt and black pepper, to taste

Directions:

Season the beef pieces with salt and pepper. In a large soup pot, heat olive oil and seal the beef in batches then set it aside in a plate, covered. Sauté the onions, mushrooms, carrots, and celery over medium high heat.

Return the meat to the pot, add water and bring to the boil. Reduce heat and simmer, covered, for about an hour, stirring occasionally. Dissolve the tomato paste in a few tablespoons of the soup broth and add it to the pot. Stir in the chopped parsley and season with salt and pepper to taste.

Beef and Vegetable Minestrone

Serves 5-6

Ingredients:

2 slices bacon, chopped

1 cup ground beef

2 carrots, chopped

2 cloves garlic, finely chopped

1 large onion, chopped

1 celery rib, chopped

1 bay leaf

1 tsp dried basil

1 tsp dried rosemary, crushed

1/4 tsp crushed chillies

1 can tomatoes, chopped

5 cups gluten-free beef broth

Directions:

In a large saucepan, cook bacon and ground beef until well done, breaking up the beef as it cooks. Drain off the fat and add carrots, garlic, onion and celery. Cook, stirring, for about 5 minutes or until the onions are translucent.

Season with the bay leaf, basil, rosemary and crushed chillies. Stir in tomatoes and beef broth. Bring to a boil then reduce heat and simmer for about 30 minutes.

Italian Meatball Soup

Serves 4-5

Ingredients:

1 lb lean ground beef

1 small onion, grated

1 onion, chopped

2 garlic cloves, crushed

1 zucchini, diced

3-4 basil leaves, finely chopped

1 egg, lightly beaten

2 cups gluten-free tomato sauce with basil

3 cups water

2 tbsp olive oil

salt and black pepper, to taste

Directions:

Combine ground beef, grated onion, garlic, basil and egg in a large bowl. Season with salt and pepper. Mix well with hands and roll tablespoonfuls of the mixture into balls. Place on a large plate.

Heat olive oil into a large deep saucepan and sauté onion and garlic until transparent. Add tomato sauce, water, and bring to the boil over high heat. Add in the meatballs. Reduce heat to medium-low and simmer, uncovered, for 10 minutes.

Meatball Soup

Serves 4-5

Ingredients:

1 lb lean ground beef

1 onion, chopped

2 garlic cloves, cut

1 tomato, diced

1 carrot, diced

1 potato, cubed

1 green pepper, chopped

3 cups water

½ bunch of parsley, finely cut

3 tbsp olive oil

½ tsp black pepper

1 tsp savory

1 tsp paprika

1 tsp salt

Directions:

Combine ground meat, savory, paprika, black pepper, and salt in a large bowl. Mix well with hands and roll teaspoonfuls of the mixture into balls. Heat olive oil into a large soup pot and sauté onion and garlic until transparent.

Add water and bring to the boil over high heat. Add the meatballs, carrot, potato and green pepper. Reduce heat to low and simmer, uncovered, for 15 minutes. Add the tomato and the parsley and cook for 5 more minutes.

Lamb Soup

Serves 4-5

Ingredients:

2 lb lean boneless lamb, cubed

1 onion, finely cut

1 carrot, chopped

4-5 spring onions, chopped

1/3 cup rice, washed and drained

1 tomato, diced

4 cups hot water

2 tbsp sunflower oil

1 tsp salt

black pepper, to taste

1 tbsp dry mint

1/2 cup parsley, finely cut

3 tbsp yogurt

1 egg

Directions:

Heat 2 tablespoonfuls of sunflower oil and gently brown the lamb cubes in a medium sized cooking pot. Add the finely cut onion and the carrot and sauté for a minute or two, stirring. Add two cups of hot water and bring to the boil, then lower heat to medium-low and simmer until the lamb softens.

Add in 2 more cups of hot water, rice, butter, green onions, tomato, mint, salt and black pepper. Bring to a boil again and simmer until the rice is done.

Whisk the the egg and the yogurt in a small bowl. Take one ladle from the soup and add into the egg mixture, whisk. Take another and whisk again. Pour this mixture back into into the soup and stir. Do not boil.

Sprinkle with parsley and serve while still hot.

Buckwheat Fish Soup

Serves 4

Ingredients:

2 lb fish steaks, cut into 1 inch pieces

4 cups water

1/3 cup buckwheat, washed

2 medium potatoes, diced

2 carrots, grated

1 medium onion, chopped

1 bay leave

1/2 cup fresh dill, chopped

lemon juice, to serve

salt and black pepper, to taste

Directions:

Place the fish, bay leave, vegetables and buckwheat groats in a pot with four cups of cold water. Bring the pot to a boil then lower heat. Simmer until fish and potatoes are done.

Season with dill, salt and black pepper just before serving. Serve with lemon juice

Chilled Celery and Prawn Soup

Serves 4-5

Ingredients:

12 cooked prawns, peeled and coarsely chopped

4 celery ribs, trimmed and chopped

2 leeks, only pale section, chopped

2 potatoes, diced

4 cups gluten-free chicken broth

1 cup coconut milk

3 tbsp sunflower oil

a pinch of cayenne pepper

1 tsp chopped fresh tarragon

Directions:

Heat the sunflower oil in a medium saucepan over medium heat. Sauté the celery and leeks, stirring, for 3-4 minutes or until the leeks are soft. Add in the potatoes, chicken broth, milk, cayenne pepper and the tarragon.

Simmer for about 30 minutes, stirring occasionally, until the potatoes are done. Set aside for 5 minutes to cool slightly.

Blend until smooth and place in the fridge until well chilled. Serve topped with the prawns.

Curried Lentil Soup

Serves 5-6

Ingredients:

1 cup dried lentils

1 large onion, finely cut

1 celery rib, chopped

1 large carrot, chopped

3 garlic cloves, chopped

1 can tomatoes, undrained

3 cups chicken broth

1 tbsp curry powder

1/2 tsp ground ginger

4 bacon slices, cooked and crumbled, to serve

Directions:

Combine all ingredients in slow cooker.

Cover and cook on low for 5-6 hours.

Blend soup to desired consistency, adding additional hot water to thin, if desired.

Serve topped with crumbled bacon.

Lemon Artichoke Soup

Serves 4-5

Ingredients:

2 cups artichoke hearts, chopped

1 small onion, very finely cut

1 celery rib, very finely cut

2 carrots, very finely cut

1 garlic clove, crushed

3 cups gluten-free chicken broth

2 tbsp olive oil

1 tsp salt

1 tsp black pepper

1 fresh lemon, halved

2 cups coconut milk

Directions:

Heat olive oil in a large pot and gently sauté onion, celery, carrot and garlic. Stir in chicken broth, artichokes, salt and pepper and bring to the boil.

Lower heat and simmer for 10 minutes. Remove from heat and blend until smooth. Return to heat, juice half a lemon into soup.

Bring to the boil, reduce heat and simmer for 5 more minutes. Stir in coconut milk and simmer for another 5 minutes.

Beetroot and Carrot Soup

Serves 6

Ingredients:

4 beets, washed and peeled

2 carrots, peeled, chopped

2 potatoes, peeled, chopped

1 medium onion, chopped

2 cups gluten-free vegetable broth

2 cups water

2 tbsp yogurt

2 tbsp olive oil

a bunch or spring onions, chopped, to serve

Directions:

Peel and chop the beets. Heat olive oil in a saucepan over medium high heat and sauté the onion and carrot until the onion is tender. Add beets, potatoes, broth and water. Bring to the boil.

Reduce heat to medium and simmer, partially covered, for 30-40 minutes, or until beets are tender. Cool slightly.

Blend soup in batches until smooth. Return it to pan over low heat and cook, stirring, for 4-5 minutes or until heated through.

Season with salt and pepper. Serve soup topped with yogurt and sprinkled with spring onions.

Minted Pea Soup

Serves 4

Ingredients:

1 onion, finely chopped

2 garlic cloves, finely chopped

3 cups gluten-free vegetable broth

1/3 cup mint leaves

2 lb green peas, frozen

3 tbsp olive oil

1/4 cup yogurt, to serve

small mint leaves, to serve

Directions:

Heat oil in a large saucepan over medium-high heat and sauté onion and garlic for 5 minutes or until soft.

Add gluten-free vegetable broth and bring to the boil, then add mint and peas. Cover, reduce heat, and cook for 3 minutes, or until peas are tender but still green. Remove from heat. Set aside to cool slightly, then blend in batches, until smooth.

Return soup to saucepan over medium-low heat and cook until heated through. Season with salt and pepper. Serve topped with yogurt, black pepper and mint leaves.

Moroccan Lentil Soup

Serves 6-7

Ingredients:

1 cup red lentils

1 cup canned chickpeas, drained

2 onions, chopped

2 cloves garlic, minced

1 cup canned tomatoes, chopped

1 cup canned white beans, drained

3 carrots, diced

3 celery ribs, diced

5 cups water

1 tsp ginger, grated

1 tsp ground cardamom

½ tsp ground cumin

3 tbsp olive oil

Directions:

In a large pot, sauté onions, garlic and ginger in olive oil, for about 5 minutes. Add the water, lentils, chickpeas, white beans, tomatoes, carrots, celery, cardamom and cumin.

Bring to a boil for a few minutes, then simmer for ½ hour or longer, until the lentils are tender.

Puree half the soup in a food processor or blender. Return the pureed soup to the pot, stir and serve.

Spinach and Mushroom Soup

Serves 4-5

Ingredients:

1 small onion, finely cut

1 small carrot, chopped

1 small zucchini, diced

2 medium potatoes, diced

5-6 white mushrooms, chopped

2 cups chopped fresh spinach

3 cups water

4 tbsp olive oil

salt and black pepper to taste

Directions:

Heat olive oil in a large pot over medium heat. Add potatoes, onions, mushrooms and water and cook until vegetables are soft but not mushy.

Add in the chopped fresh spinach, zucchini, simmer for about 15 minutes more. Season to taste with salt and pepper.

Broccoli and Potato Soup

Serves 6

Ingredients:

2 lbs broccoli, cut into florets

2 potatoes, chopped

1 big onion, chopped

3 garlic cloves, crushed

4 cups water

1 tbsp olive oil

¼ tsp ground nutmeg

Directions:

Heat oil in a large saucepan over medium-high heat. Add onion and garlic and sauté, stirring, for 3 minutes or until soft.

Add broccoli, potato and 4 cups of cold water. Cover and bring to the boil, then reduce heat to low. Simmer, stirring, for 10 to 15 minutes, or until potato is tender. Remove from heat.

Blend until smooth. Return to pan. Cook for 5 minutes or until heated through. Season with nutmeg and pepper before serving.

Leek, Rice and Potato Soup

Serves 6

Ingredients:

2-3 potatoes, diced

1 small onion, chopped

1 leek halved lengthwise and sliced

1/3 cup rice

4-5 cups of water

3 tbsp olive oil

lemon juice, to serve

Directions:

Heat a soup pot over medium heat. Add olive oil and sauté onion for 2 minutes. Add leeks and potatoes and cook for a few minutes more.

Add three cups of water, bring the soup to a boil then reduce heat and simmer for 5 minutes. Add the very well washed rice and simmer for 10 more minutes. Serve with lemon juice to taste.

Bulgarian Potato Soup

Serves 4-5

Ingredients:

1 medium onion, chopped

4-5 medium potatoes, diced

3 cups water

3 tbsp sunflower oil

1 1/2 cup whole milk

1 tsp paprika

salt, to taste

black pepper, to taste

Directions:

Heat the sunflower oil over medium heat and sauté the onion for 2-3 minutes. Add the diced potatoes and stir. Add a teaspoon of paprika and stir again.

Pour 2 cups of water and bring the soup to a boil, then lower heat and simmer until the potatoes are tender. Stir in the milk, season with salt and pepper to taste and simmer for 1-2 minutes. Serve with lemon juice to taste

Mediterranean Chickpea Soup

Serves 5-6

Ingredients:

2 cups canned chickpeas, drained

a bunch of green onions, finely cut

2 cloves garlic, crushed

1 cup canned tomatoes, diced

5 cups gluten-free vegetable broth

3 tbsp olive oil

1 bay leaf

½ tsp crushed rosemary

½ cup freshly grated Parmesan cheese

Directions:

Sauté onion and garlic in olive oil in a heavy soup pot. Add broth, chickpeas, tomato, bay leaf, and rosemary.

Bring to the boil then reduce heath and simmer for 20 minutes. Remove from heat and serve sprinkled with Parmesan cheese.

Carrot and Chickpea Soup

Serves 4-5

Ingredients:

3-4 big carrots, chopped

1 leek, chopped

4 cups gluten-free vegetable broth

1 cup canned chickpeas, undrained

½ cup orange juice

2 tbsp olive oil

½ tsp cumin

½ tsp ginger

4-5 tbsp yogurt, to serve

Directions:

Heat oil in a large saucepan over medium heat. Add leek and carrots and sauté until soft. Add orange juice, broth, chickpeas and spices.

Bring to the boil then reduce heat to medium-low and simmer, covered, for 15 minutes. Blend soup until smooth; return to pan. Season with salt and pepper. Stir over heat until heated through.

Pour in 4-5 bowls, top with yogurt and serve.

Roasted Red Pepper Soup

Serves 6-7

Ingredients:

5-6 red peppers

1 large onion, chopped

2 garlic cloves, crushed

4 medium tomatoes, chopped

4 cups gluten-free vegetable broth

3 tbsp olive oil

2 bay leaves

Directions:

Grill the peppers or roast them in the oven at 480 F until the skins are a little burnt. Place the roasted peppers in a brown paper bag or a lidded container and leave covered for about 10 minutes. This makes it easier to peel them. Peel the skins and remove the seeds. Cut the peppers in small pieces.

Heat oil in a large saucepan over medium-high heat. Add onion and garlic and sauté, stirring, for 3 minutes or until onion has softened. Add the red peppers, bay leaves, tomato and simmer for 5 minutes.

Add broth. Season with pepper. Bring to the boil then reduce heat and simmer for 20 minutes. Set aside to cool slightly. Blend, in batches, until smooth and serve.

Spring Nettle Soup

Serves 6

Ingredients:

1.5 lb young top shoots of nettles, well washed

1 cup spinach leaves

1 carrot, chopped

a bunch of spring onions, coarsely chopped

3 tbsp sunflower oil

3 cups hot water

1 tsp salt

Directions:

Clean the young nettles, wash and cook them in slightly salted water. Drain, rinse, drain again and then chop or pass through a sieve.

Sauté the chopped spring onions and carrot in the oil until the onion softens. Add in the nettles, the spinach leaves, and gradually stir in the water.

Bring to a boil, reduce heat and simmer for 5 minutes. Set aside to cool then blend in batches. Serve with a dollop of yogurt.

Gazpacho

Serves 6-7

Ingredients:

6-7 medium tomatoes, peeled and halved

1 onion, sliced

1 green pepper, sliced

1 big cucumber, peeled and sliced

2 cloves garlic

salt, to taste

4 tbsp olive oil

to garnish

1/2 onion, chopped

1 green pepper, chopped

1 cucumber, chopped

Directions:

Place the tomatoes, garlic, onion, green pepper, cucumber, salt and olive oil in a blender or food processor and puree until smooth, adding small amounts of cold water if needed to achieve desired consistency.

Serve the gazpacho chilled with the chopped onion, green pepper and cucumber.

Cold Cucumber Soup

Serves 4-5

Ingredients:

1 large or two small cucumbers

2 cups yogurt

2-3 cloves garlic, crushed or chopped

1 cup cold water

4 tbsp sunflower or olive oil

2 bunches of fresh dill, finely chopped

1/2 cup crushed walnuts

Directions:

Wash the cucumber, peel and cut it into small cubes.

In a large bowl dilute the yogurt with water to taste, add the cucumber and garlic stirring well. Add salt to the taste, garnish with the dill and the crushed walnuts and put in the fridge to cool.

Gluten-Free Main Dishes

Mediterranean Chicken Casserole

Serves 4

Ingredients:

4 chicken breast halves

1 big onion, sliced

1 red bell pepper, thinly sliced

2 cups diced tomatoes

½ cup black olives, pitted

½ green olives, pitted

1/3 cup Parmesan cheese

¼ cup chopped parsley

3 tbsp olive oil

Directions:

Heat the oil in a large, deep frying pan over medium-high heat. Cook chicken breasts, turning, for 4-5 minutes or until golden. Transfer to ovenproof casserole dish.

In the same pan, sauté the onion and bell pepper, stirring, for 3-4 minutes, or until the onion has softened. Add this mixture, together with the tomatoes and olives on and around the chicken.

Season with salt and pepper to taste and bake, in a preheated to 350 F oven, for 40 minutes. Half way through stir gently. Sprinkle with Parmesan cheese, parsley and serve.

Greek Chicken Casserole

Serves 5-6

Ingredients:

4 skinless, boneless chicken breast halves or 8 tights

2 lb potatoes, cubed

1 lb green beans, trimmed and cut in 1 inch pieces

1 big onion, chopped

1 cup diced tomatoes

5 cloves garlic, minced

1/4 cup water

½ cup feta cheese, crumbled

salt and black pepper, to taste

Directions:

Preheat oven to 350 F. Heat oil in a large baking dish over medium heat. Add onion and sauté for 2 minutes. Add thyme, black pepper and garlic and sauté for another minute. Add potatoes and sauté, for 2-3 minutes, or until they begin to brown. Stir in beans, water and tomatoes.

Remove from heat. Arrange chicken pieces into the vegetables, sprinkle with salt and pepper and top with feta. Cover and bake for 40 minutes, stirring gently halfway through. Serve the vegetable mixture on a plate underneath or beside the chicken.

Hunter Style Chicken

Serves 4-6

Ingredients:

1 chicken (about 3 lbs), cut into pieces

2 onions, thinly sliced

1-2 red bell peppers, chopped

6-7 white mushrooms, sliced

2 cups canned tomatoes, diced and drained

3 garlic cloves, thinly sliced

salt and freshly ground pepper, to taste

1/3 cup white wine

½ cup parsley leaves, finely cut

1 bay leaf

1 tsp sugar

2 tbsp olive oil

Directions:

Rinse chicken pieces and pat dry. Heat olive oil in a large skillet on medium heat. Working in batches, cook the chicken pieces until nicely browned. Transfer chicken to a bowl and set aside. Add 2 tbsp of olive oil and sauté the sliced onions and bell peppers for a few minutes. Add the mushrooms and cook some more until onion is translucent. Add in garlic and cook a minute more.

Add wine and simmer until liquid is reduced by half. Add tomatoes and a teaspoon of sugar and stir. Place chicken and the tomato mixture in an ovenproof casserole dish and bake in a preheated to 350 oven for 35-40 minutes.

Chicken with Almonds and Prunes

Serves 4

Ingredients:

1.5 lb chicken thigh fillets, trimmed

½ cup fresh orange juice

2 tbsp honey

1/3 cup white wine

½ cup pitted prunes

2 tbsp blanched almonds

2 tbsp raisins or sultanas

1 tsp ground cinnamon

salt and ground black pepper, to taste

1 tbsp fresh parsley leaves, chopped

Directions:

Combine orange juice, wine, honey, prunes, almonds, raisins and cinnamon in a large saucepan. Bring to a boil, reduce heat to medium and boil for 5-8 minutes or until liquid is reduced by 1/3.

Add the chicken thigh fillets and simmer over low heat, for 10 minutes, or until chicken is just tender. Season to taste with salt and pepper. Serve sprinkled with parsley.

Lemon Rosemary Chicken

Serves 4

Ingredients:

4 boneless skinless chicken breasts or 4-5 tights

2 garlic cloves, crushed

4-5 lemon slices

4-5 black olives, pitted

1 tbsp capers

1 tbsp dried rosemary

3 tbsp olive oil

salt and pepper, to taste

Directions:

Place the lemon slices at the bottom of a skillet and lay the chicken breasts on top of the lemon. Add in olives, rosemary, capers, salt and pepper to taste.

Cover, and cook, on medium-low, for 35-40 minutes or until the chicken is cooked through.

Uncover and cook for 2-3 minutes, until the liquid evaporates.

Chicken with Almonds and Spinach

Serves 4

Ingredients:

4 chicken breast fillets, halved

1 red bell pepper, deseeded, chopped

1 cup baby spinach leaves

1/4 cup slivered almonds

1/4 cup raisins

4 tbsp olive oil

1 tsp saffron

1 tsp nutmeg

1 tsp cinnamon

1 cup gluten-free chicken broth

½ cup quinoa

Directions:

Toss the chicken in olive oil and sprinkle with cinnamon, nutmeg and saffron. Heat a frying pan over medium heat. Add the chicken and cook for 3-4 minutes each side or until golden. Transfer to a baking dish and set aside.

In the same pan, gently sauté the bell pepper and silvered almonds, stirring, for 2 minutes. Add the raisins and cook some more. Add this mixture on and around the chicken. Add in chicken broth and quinoa and bake, in a preheated to 350 F oven, for 15 minutes or until cooked through.

Cover and set aside for 5 minutes. Fold through spinach until just wilted.

Moroccan Chicken Tagine

Serves 4-5

Ingredients:

1 whole chicken (3-4 lbs), cut into pieces

2 large onions, chopped

2-3 garlic cloves, finely chopped or pressed

½ cup green or black olives

1 preserved lemon, quartered and deseeded

5 tbsp olive oil

1 tsp grated ginger

1 tsp cumin

1 tbsp paprika

1 tsp black pepper

1 tsp turmeric

½ tsp salt

1 bunch of fresh coriander

1 bunch of fresh parsley

Directions:

Rinse and dry chicken and place onto a clean plate.

In a large bowl, mix three tablespoons of olive oil, salt, half the onions, garlic, ginger, cumin, paprika, and turmeric. Mix thoroughly, crush the garlic with your fingers, and add a little water to make a paste.

Roll the chicken pieces into the marinade and leave for 10-15 minutes.

Heat a deep casserole with a lid and add 2 tablespoons of olive oil. Add the chicken and pour excess marinade juices over the top. Add the remaining onions, olives and chopped preserved lemon. Tie the parsley and coriander together into a bouquet and place on top of the chicken.

Cover, bring to a boil and immediately reduce to a simmer. Cook for 45 minutes or until the chicken is cooked through and quite tender. Serve with rice or quinoa.

Mediterranean Chicken with Buckwheat

Serves 4-5

Ingredients:

2 chicken breast halves, cut into strips

2 garlic cloves, finely chopped

1 cup chicken broth

1 lemon, rind finely grated, juiced

1 cup buckwheat

1 cup cherry tomatoes, halved

½ cup green olives, pitted, halved

½ cup fresh parsley leaves, chopped

5-6 spring onions, trimmed, chopped

2 tbs drained capers

3 tbsp olive oil

½ tsp freshly ground black pepper

Directions:

Marinate the chicken in the oil, garlic and black pepper in a shallow dish. Heat an ovenproof casserole over medium high heat. Add half the chicken mixture and cook for 2-3 minutes, tossing, until just cooked. Transfer to a plate, cover with foil to keep warm and set aside. Repeat with the remaining chicken mixture.

Heat a large, dry saucepan and toast the buckwheat for about three minutes. Add the toasted buckwheat to the casserole together with broth and lemon juice. Add in the chicken, lemon rind, tomatoes, olives, parsley, spring onions and capers. Toss well to combine and bake in a preheated to 350 F for 15 minutes.

Chicken Moussaka

Serves 6

Ingredients:

2 big eggplants, cut into ½ inch thick rounds

olive oil cooking spray

1 tbsp salt

1 onion, finely cut

½ tsp cinnamon

½ tsp nutmeg

1/4 tsp coriander

1/4 tsp grated ginger

2 cups canned tomatoes, undrained, chopped

2 cups shredded roast chicken

½ cup finely chopped fresh parsley leaves

1 tsp sugar

1 cup yogurt

1 cup Parmesan cheese

salt and black pepper, to taste

Directions:

Place eggplant slices on a tray and sprinkle with plenty of salt. Let sit for 30 minutes, then rinse with cold water. Lay slices out flat and use a clean kitchen towel to squeeze out excess water and pat dry.

Heat a frying pan over medium high heat. Spray both sides of eggplant with oil. Cook in batches for 3-4 minutes each side or until golden. Transfer to a plate.

In the same pan sauté onion, stirring, for 3-4 minutes or until softened. Add spice. Sauté for one minute until fragrant. Add tomatoes and sugar, stir, and sauté until thickened. Add chicken and parsley and stir well to combine.

Arrange half the eggplant slices in a baking dish. Cover with chicken and tomato mixture and arrange remaining eggplant. Top with yogurt and sprinkle with Parmesan cheese. Bake for 30 minutes or until golden. Set aside for five minutes and serve.

Chicken and Artichoke Rice

Serves 4

Ingredients:

3 skinless chicken breasts, cut into strips

2 leeks, white parts only, chopped

4-5 char-grilled artichokes hearts, quartered

2 garlic cloves, crushed

1/3 cup rice

1 cup chicken broth

2 tbsp olive oil

1 tsp lemon rind

7-8 fresh basil leaves, chopped

1 bay leaf

juice of 1 lemon

Directions:

Heat the oil in a large saucepan over low heat. Gently sauté the leeks, bay leaf and garlic for about 3-4 minutes, stirring occasionally. Add in the lemon rind and the chicken breasts and cook, stirring, for 5-6 minutes.

Add rice, stir, and add chicken broth and half the lemon juice. Bring to the boil, then reduce heat, cover, and cook for 10 minutes. Set aside covered for 5 minutes then stir in the chopped basil, artichokes hearts and remaining lemon juice.

Easy Chicken Parmigiana

Serves 4

Ingredients:

4 chicken breast fillets

1 eggplant, peeled and sliced lengthwise

1 can tomatoes, diced

9 oz mozzarella cheese, sliced

2 tbsp olive oil

Directions:

Place chicken into an ovenproof casserole. Heat olive oil in a non-stick frying pan and cook eggplant in batches, for 1-2 minutes each side, or until golden. Place eggplant over the chicken and add in tomatoes.

Top with mozzarella slices and bake, in a preheated to 350 F, for 20 minutes, or until the cheese is golden.

Sweet and Sour Sicilian Chicken

Serves 4

Ingredients:

4 chicken thigh fillets

1 large red onion, sliced

3 garlic cloves, chopped

1/3 cup dry white wine

1 cup chicken broth

½ cup green olives

2 tbsp olive oil

2 bay leaves

1 tbsp fresh oregano leaves

2 tbsp brown sugar or honey

2 tbsp red wine vinegar

salt and black pepper, to taste

Directions:

Sprinkle the chicken pieces with salt and black pepper. Heat oil in a large non-stick frying pan and cook the chicken in batches, for 1-2 minutes each side, or until golden. Transfer to a baking dish.

In the same pan, gently sauté the onion and garlic, stirring, for 2 minutes or until soft. Add in the wine and cook for 1 minute. Add the chicken broth, olives, bay leaves, oregano, sugar and vinegar and bring to the boil. Simmer for 3-4 minutes then pour over the chicken. Bake, in a preheated to 380 F oven, for 20 minutes, or until the chicken is cooked through.

Mediterranean Beef Casserole

Serves 6

Ingredients:

2 lb lean steak, cut into large pieces

3 onions, sliced

4 garlic cloves, cut

2 red peppers, cut

1 green pepper, cut

1 zucchini, cut

3 tomatoes, quartered

2 tbsp tomato paste or purée

½ cup green olives, pitted

½ cup dry red wine

½ cup of water

1 tsp dry oregano

salt and black pepper, to taste

Directions:

Heat olive oil in a deep ovenproof casserole and seal the beef. Add vegetables and stir. Dilute the tomato paste in half a cup of water and pour it over the meat mixture together with the wine.

Season well and bake, stirring halfway through, in a preheated to 350 F for one hour.

Ground Beef and Chickpea Casserole

Serves 4-5

Ingredients:

1 lb ground beef

1 onion, chopped

2 garlic cloves, crushed

1 can chickpeas, drained

1 can sweet corn, drained

1 can gluten-free tomato sauce

½ cup water

2 bay leaves

1 tsp dried oregano

½ tsp salt

½ tsp cumin

3 tbsp olive oil

black pepper, to taste

Directions:

Heat the olive oil in an ovenproof casserole over medium-high heat. Add the onion and sauté for 4-5 minutes. Add garlic and sauté a minute more. Add in the ground beef and cook for 5 minutes, stirring, until browned. Add the cumin and bay leaves, the tomatoes, corn and chickpeas.

Bake in a preheated to 350 F for 20 minutes, or until the beef is cooked through. Remove the bay leaves and serve.

Ground Beef and Rice Stuffed Peppers

Serves 6

Ingredients:

6 red or green bell peppers, cored and seeded

1 lb ground beef

1/4 cup rice, washed and drained

1 onion, finely cut

1 small tomato, grated

a bunch of fresh parsley, chopped

3 tbsp olive oil

1 tbsp paprika

salt and black pepper, to taste

Directions:

Heat the oil and gently sauté the onion for 2-3 minutes. Remove from heat. Add paprika, ground beef, rice and grated tomato, and season with salt and pepper. Combine ingredients very well and stuff each pepper with the mixture using a spoon. Every pepper should be 3/4 full.

Arrange the peppers in a deep ovenproof dish and top up with warm water to half fill the dish. Cover with a lid or foil and bake for about 40 minutes at 350 F. Uncover and bake for 5 minutes more. Serve with yogurt.

Potato Moussaka

Serves 4

Ingredients:

1 lb ground beef

1 celery rib, finely chopped

1 carrot, peeled, finely chopped

1 onion, finely chopped

2 garlic cloves, crushed

1 cup canned tomatoes, drained, diced

5 potatoes, cut into 1/4 inch cubes

½ cup fresh parsley leaves, finely cut

3 tbsp olive oil

1 tbsp summer savory

1 tsp paprika

2/3 cup yogurt

1 egg, lightly beaten

salt and freshly ground black pepper, to taste

Directions:

Heat half the oil in a large frying pan over medium-high heat. Add the ground meat and cook, stirring, using a spoon to break up lumps, for 5 minutes or until it changes color. Transfer to a large baking dish.

Heat the remaining oil in the same pan. Add the carrot, onion, garlic, parsley, paprika and savory and sauté, stirring, for 10 minutes, or until vegetables soften. Transfer to the baking dish and mix well with ground meat.

Wash, peel, and cut into small 1/4 inch cubes the potatoes. Stir potatoes into the meat and the vegetable mixture. Combine very well, add ½ cup of water, stir again and bake in a preheated to 350 F oven for 30 minutes, or until potatoes are cooked through.

In a small bowl, mix together the yogurt and egg, pour and spread it evenly over the Moussaka. Bake for 5 more minutes or until golden. Set aside for five minutes and serve with a dollop of yogurt.

Eggplant Moussaka

Serves 6

Ingredients:

1 ½ lbs ground beef

3 eggplants, peeled and cut into ½ inch thick rounds

1 big onion, chopped

½ tsp cinnamon

1/4 tsp coriander

½ cup canned tomatoes, undrained, chopped

½ cup parsley leaves, finely chopped

4 tbsp olive oil

1 tsp sugar

1 tsp salt

2/3 cup yogurt

1 egg

1 cup Parmesan cheese

salt and black pepper, to taste

Directions:

Place eggplant rounds on a tray and sprinkle with plenty of salt. Let sit for 30 minutes, then rinse with cold water. Squeeze out excess water and pat dry.

Heat oil in a frying pan over medium high heat. Cook eggplant, in batches, for 3 to 4 minutes each side, or until golden. Transfer to a plate.

softened. Add spice and sauté for one more minute until fragrant. Add ground beef, garlic, sugar and tomatoes. Stir and cook until the meat is no longer pink.

Arrange half the eggplant slices in a baking dish. Cover with meat mixture and arrange remaining eggplant. Bake in a preheated to 350 F oven for 30 minutes.

In a small bowl mix together the yogurt, egg, and Parmesan cheese, pour and spread it evenly over the Moussaka. Bake for 5 more minutes, or until golden. Set aside for five minutes and serve.

Zucchini Moussaka

Serves 4

Ingredients:

1 lb ground beef

4-5 zucchinis, sliced

1/3 cup rice

3-4 garlic cloves, sliced

1 large onion, chopped

½ cup canned tomatoes

½ cup fresh dill, finely cut

2/3 cup yogurt

1 egg, lightly beaten

4 tbsp olive oil

1 tsp paprika

salt and black pepper, to taste

Directions:

Sauté the onions and garlic for a minute or two, stirring. Add the ground beef and cook it for 10 minutes until it is no longer pink. Add tomatoes, paprika, rice and dill and stir. Arrange half the zucchini slices in a baking pan. Spread ground beef mixture over them. Arrange the remaining zucchinis on top. Bake in a preheated to 350 F oven for 30 minutes.

In a small bowl, mix together the yogurt and egg, pour and spread it evenly over the Zucchini Moussaka. Bake for 5 more minutes, or until golden. Set aside for five minutes and serve.

Mediterranean Lamb Casserole

Serves 5

Ingredients:

2 lb boned lean shoulder of lamb

3 onions, sliced

2 garlic cloves, chopped

1 15 oz can chickpeas, drained and rinsed

2 zucchinis, peeled and cubed

1 cup cherry tomatoes, halved

1 cup beef broth

1 cup tomato juice

3 tbsp olive oil

1 tbsp fresh rosemary, chopped

1 tbsp fresh basil, chopped

½ cup fresh parsley leaves, to serve

Directions:

Cut the lamb into 1 inch cubes. In an ovenproof casserole, heat 2 tablespoons of the olive oil and gently sauté onions and garlic for about 2-3 minutes. Add the lamb and sauté, stirring, for about 4 minutes or until well browned on all sides.

Add in rosemary, tomato juice and beef broth and bake in a preheated to 350 F for 1 hour.

Stir in the chickpeas and bake for a further 1 hour or until the lamb is almost tender. Stir in zucchinis, tomatoes, black pepper and basil. Cook for about 20 minutes longer or until the lamb is tender. Serve sprinkled with parsley.

Lamb and Potato Casserole

Serves 6

Ingredients:

2 pounds shoulder lamb chops

15 small new potatoes, peeled, whole

3 large onions, sliced

2 carrots, sliced

2 tbsp olive oil

2 tsp dried parsley

2 tsp dried mint

½ tsp black pepper

½ tsp salt

Directions:

Place the lamb chops into a greased casserole dish. Cover them with sliced onion, carrots, parsley, salt and pepper.

Arrange new potatoes on and around the meat. Add enough cold water to fill the dish halfway.

Bake, covered with foil, for 45 minutes in a preheated oven. Remove the foil and bake for 30 minutes more.

Spring Lamb Casserole

Serves 6

Ingredients:

1 1/2 lb lamb meat, cubed

1 lb mushrooms, chopped

1 onion, cut

2 bunches fresh spring onions, cut

2 tomatoes, chopped

3 tbsp olive oil

1 tsp paprika

a bunch of fresh mint, finely cut

2 bunches of fresh parsley, finely cut

Directions:

Heat olive oil in an ovenproof casserole. Sauté the lamb pieces until browned. Add in onions and cook some more. Add paprika, cover with foil or a lid and bake at 350 F for an hour or until tender.

Add in spring onions, mushrooms, tomatoes, mint and parsley and bake, uncovered, for 10 more minutes or until the liquid evaporates.

Mediterranean Pork Casserole

Serves 5

Ingredients:

2 lb pork loin, cut into cubes

1 large onion, chopped

1 cup mushrooms, cut

½ cup chicken broth

2 garlic cloves, finely chopped

1 green pepper, deseeded and cut into strips

1 red pepper, deseeded and cut into strips

1 tomato, chopped

2 tsp olive oil

1 tsp summer savory

1 tsp paprika

salt and black pepper, to taste

Directions:

Add the olive oil to a casserole dish and seal the pork cubes for about 5 minutes, stirring continuously. Lower the heat, add the onion and garlic and sauté for 3-4 minutes until the onion is soft.

Add the paprika and summer savory and season with salt and pepper to taste. Stir in the peppers, tomato, chicken broth and mushrooms.

Cover with a lid or foil, and bake for 1 hour at 350 F, or until the pork is tender. Uncover and bake for 5 minutes more. Serve with boiled potatoes.

Pork and Mushroom Casserole

Serves 5

Ingredients:

2 lb pork loin, cut into cubes

1 large onion, chopped

1 carrot, chopped

2 cups mushrooms, cut

3 tbsp olive oil

1/3 cup sour cream

salt and black pepper, to taste

Directions:

Heat the olive oil in a casserole dish and seal the pork cubes for about 5 minutes, stirring continuously. Lower the heat, add the onion and carrot and sauté for 3-4 minutes until the onion is soft.

Cover wit a lid or foil and simmer for 1 hour at 350 F, or until the pork is tender. Uncover, add the sour cream, salt and pepper to taste, stir, and bake for 10 minutes more. Serve with boiled potatoes or gluten-free pasta.

Pork and Rice Casserole

Serves 4

Ingredients:

1.5 lb pork, cubed (leg or neck)

1 onion, cut

1 1/2 cup rice, washed

4 cups water

4 tbsp olive oil

½ cup finely cut parsley leaves, to serve

Directions:

Cut pork into pieces - approximately 2x1.2 inch. Heat two tablespoons of oil in a large, deep, frying pan over medium-high heat. Cook pork, turning, for 4-5 minutes, or until browned.

Transfer to an ovenproof baking dish.

In the same pan, heat the remaining oil and sauté onion for 2-3 minutes. Add washed and drained rice and cook for 2-3 minutes, stirring continuously, until transparent.

Transfer to the baking dish. Add 5 cups of warm water, stir well and bake in a preheated to 350 F oven for 40 minutes, stirring halfway through. When ready, sprinkle with parsley, set aside for 2-3 minutes and serve.

Pork Roast and Cabbage

Serves 4

Ingredients:

2 cups of cooked pork roast, chopped

1/2 head of cabbage, chopped

2 onions, chopped

1 lemon, juice only

1 tomato, chopped

1 tsp paprika

1/2 tsp cumin

black pepper, to taste

2 tbsp olive oil

Directions:

Heat olive oil in an ovenproof casserole and sauté cabbage, pork and onions.

Add cumin, paprika, lemon juice, tomato and stir. Cover and bake at 350 F until vegetables are tender.

Mediterranean Baked Fish

Serves 4

Ingredients:

1 ½ flounder or sole fillets

3 tomatoes, chopped

½ onion, chopped

2 cloves garlic, chopped

1/3 cup white wine

20 black olives, pitted and chopped

3 tbsp olive oil

1 tbsp fresh lemon juice

4-5 fresh oregano leaves

6-7 leaves fresh basil, chopped

3 tbsp Parmesan cheese

Directions:

Preheat oven to 350 F. Heat olive oil in an ovenproof casserole and sauté onion until translucent. Add in garlic, oregano and tomatoes. Stir and cook for 4-5 minutes. Add wine, olives, lemon juice and chopped basil.

Blend in Parmesan cheese and arrange fish in this sauce. Bake for 20 minutes in the preheated oven, until fish is easily flaked with a fork.

Sea Bass Baked with Fennel

Serves 4

Ingredients:

4 skinned sea bass fillets, 4½ oz each

5 oz fennel, trimmed and sliced

½ cup dry white wine

a bunch of green onions, chopped

10 black olives, pitted and halved

1 tbsp lemon zest

2 garlic cloves, finely chopped

1 tsp paprika

salt and pepper, to taste

Directions:

Arrange the sliced fennel in a shallow ovenproof casserole. Add the green onions and lay the fish on top. Season with salt and pepper to taste. Scatter the garlic, olives, paprika and lemon zest over the fish, then pour the wine over the top.

Cover the dish with foil and bake for 30 minutes, or until the fish flakes easily.

Ratatouille

Serves 4

Ingredients:

1 eggplant, peeled and cut into small cubes

2 large tomatoes, chopped

2 zucchinis, peeled and sliced into rings

1 onion, sliced into rings

1 green pepper, sliced

6-7 sliced fresh mushrooms

3 cloves garlic, crushed

2 tsp dried parsley

½ cup Parmesan cheese

3 tbsp olive oil

Directions:

Place eggplant pieces on a tray and sprinkle with plenty of salt. Let sit for 30 minutes, then rinse with cold water.

Heat olive oil in an ovenproof casserole over medium heat. Gently sauté garlic for a minute or two. Add in parsley and eggplant. Continue sautéing until eggplant is soft. Sprinkle with a tablespoon of Parmesan cheese.

Spread the zucchinis in an even layer over the eggplant. Sprinkle with a little more cheese.

Continue layering onion, mushrooms, pepper and tomatoes, covering each layer with a sprinkling of Parmesan cheese. Bake in a preheated to 350 F oven for 40 minutes.

Spinach, Lentil and Quinoa Casserole

Serves 6

Ingredients:

½ cup brown lentils

½ cup quinoa

3 cups fresh spinach or about half package of frozen spinach, thawed

1 onion, chopped

2 medium carrots, chopped

2 cloves garlic, cut

3 tbsp olive oil

1 tbsp paprika

2 tsp summer savory

2 cups water

salt and black pepper, to taste

Directions:

Heath the olive oil in a deep casserole dish and gently sauté the onion and carrots for 4-5 minutes. Add in garlic, paprika, savory and lentils and sauté for a minute more while stirring.

Stir in the water and bake at 350 F for 15 minutes. Wash and rinse the quinoa and add it to the casserole with salt and pepper to taste. Stir well and bake for another 10 minutes. Cut the spinach and add it to casserole dish. Bake for 4-5 more minutes and serve.

Eggplant Casserole

Serves 4

Ingredients:

2 medium eggplants, peeled and diced

1 cup canned tomatoes, drained and diced

1 zucchini, diced

9-10 black olives, pitted

1 onion, chopped

4 garlic cloves, chopped

2 tbsp tomato paste

1 cup canned tomatoes, drained and diced

1 bunch of parsley, chopped, to serve

3 tbsp olive oil

1 tbsp paprika

salt and black pepper, to taste

Directions:

Heat olive oil in a deep casserole dish and gently sauté onions, garlic, and eggplants. Add in paprika and tomato paste and sauté, stirring, for 1-2 minutes.

Add in the rest of the ingredients. Cover and bake at 350 F for 30-40 minutes. Sprinkle with parsley and serve.

Eggplant and Chickpea Casserole

Serves 4

Ingredients:

2-3 eggplants, peeled and diced

1 onion, chopped

2-3 garlic cloves, crushed

1 can chickpeas, (15 oz), drained

1 can tomatoes, (15 oz), undrained, diced

1 tsp paprika

½ tsp cinnamon

1 tsp cumin

4 tbsp olive oil

salt and pepper, to taste

1 cup grated Parmesan cheese

Directions:

Peel and dice the eggplants. Heat olive oil in a deep ovenproof casserole and sauté onions and crushed garlic. Add paprika, cumin and cinnamon. Stir well to coat evenly. Sauté for 3-4 minutes until the onions have softened.

Add the eggplant, tomatoes and chickpeas. Bake in a preheated to 350 F oven, covered, for 15 minutes, or until the eggplant is tender. Uncover and sprinkle with Parmesan cheese. Bake for a few more minutes until the liquid evaporates and the cheese is golden.

Green Pea and Mushroom Stew

Serves 4

Ingredients:

1 cup green peas (fresh or frozen)

4 large mushrooms, sliced

3 spring onions, chopped

1-2 cloves garlic

4 tbsp olive oil

½ cup water

½ bunch of finely chopped dill

Directions:

In a ovenproof casserole sauté mushrooms, green onions and garlic. Add green peas and water and bake at 350 F for 20 minutes until tender. When ready sprinkle with dill and serve warm.

Cabbage and Rice Stew

Serves 4

Ingredients:

1 cup long grain white rice

2 cups water

2 tbsp olive oil

1 small onion, chopped

1 clove garlic, crushed

½ head cabbage, cored and shredded

2 tomatoes, diced

1 tbsp paprika

1 tsp cumin

salt, to taste

black pepper, to taste

½ bunch of parsley, finely cut

Directions:

Heat the olive oil in a large ovenproof casserole. Add in onion and garlic and cook until transparent. Add paprika, cumin, rice and water, stir, and bring to a boil.

Simmer for 10 minutes. Add the shredded cabbage; tomatoes, and bake in a preheated to 350 F oven for about 20 minutes, stirring occasionally, until the cabbage cooks down. Season with salt and pepper and serve sprinkled with fresh parsley.

Rice with Leeks and Olives

Serves 4-6

Ingredients:

6 large leeks, cleaned and sliced into bite sized pieces (about 6-7 cups of sliced leeks)

1 large onion, chopped

20 black olives pitted, chopped

½ cup hot water

4-5 tbsp olive oil

1 cup rice

2 cups boiling water

freshly-ground black pepper, to taste

Directions:

In a large casserole, sauté the leeks and onion in olive oil for 4-5 minutes. Add in the olives, rice and water; season with salt and black pepper.

Stir to combine and bake in a preheated to 350 F oven for 20 minutes.

Potato and Zucchini Bake

Serves 6

Ingredients:

1½ lb potatoes, peeled and sliced into rounds

4-5 zucchinis, sliced into rounds

2 onions, sliced into rounds

3 tomatoes, pureed

½ cup water

4 tbsp olive oil

1 tsp dry oregano

1/3 cup fresh parsley leaves, chopped

salt and black pepper, to taste

Directions:

Place the potatoes, zucchinis and onions in a large, shallow ovenproof baking dish. Pour over the the olive oil and pureed tomatoes.

Add salt and freshly ground pepper to taste and toss the everything together. Add in the water.

Bake in a preheated to 350 F oven for an hour, stirring halfway through.

Okra and Tomato Casserole

Serves 4-5

Ingredients:

1 lb okra, stem ends trimmed

4 large tomatoes, cut into wedges

3 garlic cloves, chopped

3 tbsp olive oil

1 tsp salt

black pepper, to taste

Directions:

In a large casserole, mix together trimmed okra, sliced tomatoes, olive oil and the chopped garlic.

Add salt and pepper and toss to combine. Bake in a preheated to 350 F oven for 45 minutes, or until the okra is tender.

Gluten-Free Breakfasts and Desserts

Winter Greens Smoothie

Serves: 2

Prep time: 5 min

Ingredients:

2 broccoli florets, frozen

1½ cup coconut water

½ banana

½ cup pineapple

1 cup fresh spinach

2 kale leaves

Directions:

Combine ingredients in blender and blend until smooth. Enjoy!

Pineapple Smoothie

Serves: 2

Prep time: 5 min

Ingredients:

2-3 ice cubes

2-3 oranges, juiced

2 cups pineapple, chopped

1 carrot, chopped

1 tbsp ground pumpkin seeds

1 tsp grated ginger

Directions:

Juice the oranges then combine with ice, carrot and pineapple in a blender. Add the pumpkin seeds ginger and blend until smooth. Enjoy!

Kiwi and Pear Smoothie

Serves: 2

Prep time: 5 min

Ingredients:

1 frozen banana, chopped

3 oranges, juiced

2 kiwi, peeled and halved

1 pear, chopped

1 tbsp coconut butter

Directions:

Juice oranges and combine all ingredients in a blender then blend until smooth. Enjoy!

Quinoa Banana Pudding

Serves 4

Ingredients:

1 cup quinoa

2 cups water

3 ripe bananas

4 cups water

4 tbsp sugar

1 tsp vanilla extract

Directions:

Wash and cook quinoa according to package directions. When ready remove from heat and set aside. In a separate bowl blend sugar and bananas until smooth. Add to the quinoa.

Heat over medium heat, string until creamy. Stir in vanilla and serve warm.

Raisin Quinoa Breakfast

Serves 2

Ingredients:

½ cup quinoa

1 cup water

1 tsp cinnamon

½ tsp vanilla

½ tsp ground flax seed

2 tbsp walnuts or almonds, chopped

2 tbsp raisins

3-4 tbsp pure maple syrup

Directions:

Rinse quinoa and drain. Place water and quinoa into a small saucepan and bring to a boil. Add cinnamon and vanilla. Reduce heat to low and simmer for about 15 minutes stirring often.

When ready, place a portion of the quinoa into a bowl, drizzle with maple syrup and top with flax seeds, raisins and crushed walnuts.

Berry Quinoa Breakfast

Serves 2

Ingredients:

½ cup quinoa

1 cup water

¼ cup fresh blueberries or raspberries

1 tbsp walnuts or almonds, chopped

3-4 tbsp pure maple syrup

1 tbsp chia seeds

Directions:

Wash quinoa and cook according to package directions. When ready, add walnuts and cinnamon, place a portion of the quinoa into a bowl and top with fresh blueberries, chia seeds and maple syrup.

Baked Apples

Serves 4

Ingredients:

8 medium sized apples

1/3 cup walnuts, crushed

3/4 cup sugar

3 tbsp raisins, soaked

vanilla, cinnamon according to taste

Directions:

Peel and carefully hollow the apples. Prepare stuffing by mixing 3/4 cup of sugar, crushed walnuts, raisins and cinnamon. Stuff the apples and place in an oiled dish, pour over 1-2 tbsp of water and bake in a moderate oven. Serve warm.

Pumpkin with Dry Fruit

Serves 5-6

Ingredients:

1.5 lb pumpkin, cut into medium pieces

1 cup dry fruit (apricots, plums, apples, raisins)

½ cup brown sugar

Directions:

Soak the dry fruit in some water, drain and discard the water. Cut the pumpkin in medium cubes. At the bottom of a pot arrange a layer of pumpkin pieces, then a layer of dry fruit and then again some pumpkin. Add a little water.

Cover the pot and bring to boil. Simmer until there is no more water left. When almost ready add the sugar. Serve warm or cold.

FREE BONUS RECIPES: Superfood Gluten-free and Vegan Smoothies for Vibrant Health and Easy Weight Loss

Peach and Cucumber Smoothie

Serves: 2

Prep time: 5 min

Ingredients:

1 frozen banana, chopped

1 cup almond milk

2 peaches, sliced

1 small cucumber, peeled

1 tsp chia seeds

Directions:

Combine ingredients in a blender and purée until smooth. Enjoy!

Antioxidant Allium Smoothie

Serves: 2

Prep time: 5 min

Ingredients:

2-3 frozen broccoli florets

1 cup water

½ avocado

1 apple, cut

½ leek

1 celery rid, cut

1 garlic clove

a pinch of salt

Directions:

Combine ingredients in a blender and purée until smooth. Enjoy!

Strawberry and Asparagus Smoothie

Serves: 2

Prep time: 5 min

Ingredients:

1 cup orange juice

1 cup frozen strawberries

½ banana, chopped

½ cup raw asparagus, chopped

3-4 dates

Directions:

Combine ingredients in a blender and purée until smooth. Enjoy!

Mango and Asparagus Smoothie

Serves: 2

Prep time: 5 min

Ingredients:

1 frozen banana, chopped

1 cup water or green tea

1 mango, peeled and chopped

½ cup raw asparagus, chopped

1 lime, juiced

1 tsp sesame seeds

Directions:

Combine ingredients in a blender and purée until smooth. Enjoy!

Pineapple and Asparagus Smoothie

Serves: 2

Prep time: 5 min

Ingredients:

2-3 ice cubes

1 cup apple juice

1 pear, cut

½ cup raw asparagus, chopped

½ cup pineapple, chopped

2-3 mint leaves

Directions:

Combine ingredients in a blender and purée until smooth. Enjoy!

Fennel and Kale Smoothie

Serves: 2

Prep time: 5 min

Ingredients:

1-2 ice cubes

1 cup coconut water

1 cup fennel

2-3 kale leaves

2-3 fresh figs

2 limes, juiced

Directions:

Combine ingredients in a blender and purée until smooth. Enjoy!

Kids' Favorite Kale Smoothie

Serves: 2

Prep time: 5 min

Ingredients:

2-3 ice cubes

1½ cup apple juice

1 small apple, cut

½ cup pineapple chunks

½ cucumber, cut

3 leaves kale

Directions:

Combine ingredients in a blender and purée until smooth. Enjoy!

Kids' Favorite Spinach Smoothie

Serves: 2

Prep time: 5 min

Ingredients:

1 frozen banana

1 cup orange juice

1 apple, cut

1 cup baby spinach

1 tsp vanilla extract

Directions:

Combine ingredients in a blender and purée until smooth. Enjoy!

Paleo Mojito Smoothie

Serves: 2

Prep time: 5 min

Ingredients:

1 cup ice

1 cup coconut water, milk or plain water

1 big pear, chopped

2-3 limes, juiced, or peeled and cut

20-25 leaves fresh mint

3 dates, pitted

Directions:

Juice the limes or peel and cut them and combine with the other ingredients in a blender. Process until smooth. Enjoy!

Winter Greens Smoothie

Serves: 2

Prep time: 5 min

Ingredients:

2 broccoli florets, frozen

1½ cup coconut water

½ banana

½ cup pineapple

1 cup fresh spinach

2 kale leaves

Directions:

Combine ingredients in blender and blend until smooth. Enjoy!

Delicious Kale Smoothie

Serves: 2

Prep time: 5 min

Ingredients:

2-3 ice cubes

1½ cup apple juice

3-4 kale leaves

1 apple, cut

1 cup strawberries

½ tsp cloves

Directions:

Combine ingredients in blender and purée until smooth.

Cherry Smoothie

Serves: 2

Prep time: 5 min

Ingredients:

2-3 ice cubes

1½ cup almond or coconut milk

1½ cup pitted and frozen cherries

½ avocado

1 tsp cinnamon

1 tsp chia seeds

Directions :

Combine all ingredients into a blender and process until smooth. Enjoy!

Banana and Coconut Smoothie

Serves: 2

Prep time: 5 min

Ingredients:

1 frozen banana, chopped

1½ cup coconut water

2-3 small broccoli florets

1 tbsp coconut butter

Directions :

Add all ingredients into a blender and blend until the smoothie turns into an even and smooth consistency. Enjoy!

Avocado and Pineapple Smoothie

Serves: 2

Prep time: 5 min

Ingredients:

3-4 ice cubes

1½ cup coconut water

½ avocado

2 cups diced pineapple

Directions:

Combine all ingredients in a blender, and blend until smooth. Enjoy!

Carrot and Mango Smoothie

Serves: 2

Prep time: 5 min

Ingredients:

1 cup frozen mango chunks

1 cup carrot juice

½ cup orange juice

1 carrot, chopped

1 tsp chia seeds

1 tsp grated ginger

Directions:

Combine all ingredients in a blender, and blend until smooth. Enjoy!

Strawberry and Coconut Smoothie

Serves: 2

Prep time: 5 min

Ingredients:

3-4 ice cubes

1½ cup coconut milk

2 cups fresh strawberries

1 tsp chia seeds

Directions:

Place all ingredients in a blender and purée until smooth. Enjoy!

Beautiful Skin Smoothie

Serves: 2

Prep time: 5 min

Ingredients:

1 cup frozen strawberries

1½ cup green tea

1 peach, chopped

½ avocado

5-6 raw almonds

1 tsp coconut oil

Directions:

Place all ingredients in a blender and purée until smooth. Enjoy!

About the Author

Vesela lives in Bulgaria with her family of six (including the Jack Russell Terrier). Her passion is going green in everyday life and she loves to prepare homemade cosmetic and beauty products for all her family and friends.

Vesela has been publishing her cookbooks for over a year now. If you want to see other healthy family recipes that she has published, together with some natural beauty books, you can check out her [Author Page](#) on Amazon.

Made in the USA
Columbia, SC
03 March 2022